Copyright 2023

Table of Contents

Pulmonary fibrosis is a serious, lifelong lung disease. It causes lung scarring (tissues scar and thicken over time), making it harder to breathe. Symptoms may come on quickly or take years to develop. No cure exists. Medications may slow down scarring and help preserve lung function. Oxygen therapy and staying active may relieve symptoms.

BREAKFAST

1. Skillet Pumpkin Cake (Gluten Free + Vegan)

Prep Time: 10Minutes

Cook Time: 25Minutes

Servings: 6

Ingredients

For The Crumble Topping:

- 3/4 cup walnuts or pecan, chopped
- 3 tbsp almond flour
- 3 tbsp coconut sugar
- 1/2 tsp cinnamon powder (I prefer Ceylon cinnamon)
- Pinch of salt
- 2 tbsp coconut oil, melted

For Skillet Pumpkin Cake:

- 1 and 3/4 cup gluten free oat flour (see note)
- 1/2 cup almond flour
- 1/3 cup coconut sugar

- 1 and 1/2 tsp baking powder
- 1/2 tsp baking soda
- 2 tsp pumpkin pie spice
- 1/2 tsp salt
- 1 cup pumpkin puree
- 1 flax eggs (1 tbsp ground flax meal + 2 and 1/2 tbsp warm water)
- 1/3 cup maple syrup
- 1/4 cup coconut oil, melted
- 1 tsp vanilla extract

Instructions

1. Preheat oven to 350'F. Liberally grease a 10 inch skillet.
2. Start by making flax egg: whisk together 1 tablespoon of ground flax meal and 2 and 1/2 tablespoons of warm water. Set aside to gel for 5 minutes.
3. Make crumble topping in a small bowl by combining nuts, almond flour, coconut sugar, cinnamon, and salt. Drizzle melted coconut oil over top and mix until well incorporated. Set aside.

4. To make cake, in a large bowl, combine oat flour, almond flour, coconut sugar, baking powder, baking soda, pumpkin pie spice, and salt.

5. In another bowl, whisk together pumpkin puree, flax egg, maple syrup, coconut oil, and vanilla extract. Stir wet ingredients into dry until well incorporated.

6. Spread cake batter into prepared skillet. Sprinkle crumble topping evenly over top.

7. Bake for 30-35 minutes, until golden and toothpick comes out clean in center. Allow to cool before slicing.

Prep Time: 15Minutes

Cook Time: 40Minutes

Servings: 9

Ingredients:

For Apple Topping:

- 1/2 cup apples, peeled and chopped
- 1 tbsp coconut sugar
- 1/2 tsp cinnamon powder

For Apple Cake Bars:

- 2 tbsp ground flax seeds
- 5 tbsp warm water
- 1 cup gluten free oat flour
- 3/4 cup almond flour
- 1 and 1/2 tsp baking powder
- 1/2 tsp baking soda
- 1 tsp cinnamon powder
- 1/4 tsp ginger powder
- 1/4 tsp cardamom or allspice
- 1/2 tsp salt

- 1/2 cup unsweetened apple sauce

- 1/4 cup coconut oil, melted

- 1/2 cup coconut sugar

- 1 tsp vanilla extract

- 1 cup apples, peeled and chopped

For Maple Glaze:

- 1/4 cup coconut butter

- 1 tbsp coconut oil

- 1 tbsp maple syrup

- Hot water

Instructions

1. Preheat oven to 350'F. Line an 8×8 pan with parchment paper.

2. To make apple topping, combine 1/2 cup chopped apples with coconut sugar and cinnamon. Set aside.

3. To make flax eggs, whisk together flax meal and warm water. Set aside for 5 minutes to gel.

4. In a medium bowl, combine oat flour, almond flour, baking powder, baking soda, spices, and salt.

5. In a large bowl. Whisk together apple sauce, coconut oil, coconut sugar, and vanilla extract. Whisk in flax

eggs. Add dry mixture to wet and stir until well incorporated. Fold in 1 cup of chopped apples.

6. Pour mixture into prepared baking pan. Spread apple topping over the top of mixture. Bake for 35-40 minutes until edges are golden and toothpick comes out clean in center.

7. Cool for 10 minutes in pan then then transfer to a wire rack to cool completely before adding maple glaze.

8. When apple bread bars are cool, prepare glaze by melting coconut butter and coconut oil in a small double boiler (I place a small glass bowl over a small pot). Whisk in 1 tablespoon of maple syrup. Taste and add more sweetener if necessary. Don't worry if it gets clumpy. Remove from heat and whisk in hot water 1 teaspoon at a time until glaze is smooth and glossy. Keep whisking. It will get there.

9. Once glaze is creamy, smooth, and thin enough to drip, drizzle or spoon over bars. Allow glaze to harden before cutting into 9 even-sized bars.

Prep Time: 15 Minutes

Cook Time: 40 Minutes

Servings: 9

Ingredients

- 3/4 cup nut or seed butter (I used tahini)
- 1/4 cup maple syrup
- 1 tsp vanilla extract
- 1 and 1/2 cups gluten free rolled oats
- 1/3 cup nuts and/or seeds (I used a combo of pumpkins seeds and sunflower seeds)
- 1/4 cup unsweetened shredded coconut
- 3 tbsp flax meal
- 2 tbsp chia seeds
- 1/4 tsp cardamom (or cinnamon)
- 1/4 tsp salt
- 1/3 cup mini chocolate chips (I use THESE sugar free chips)
- 1/3 cup dried raspberries, roughly chopped

Instructions

1. Line a baking tray with parchment paper.
2. In a large bowl, whisk together nut/seeds butter, maple syrup, and vanilla extract. Set aside.
3. In a food processor, combine oats, nuts/seeds, coconut shreds, flax meal, chia seeds, cardamom, and salt. Pulse several times until oats broken up but not powdery.
4. Add oat mixture to wet mixture in the large bowl. Mix until well incorporated. I use my hands here. Then fold in chocolate chips and dried raspberries.
5. Roll into balls and place into prepared baking sheet. Using a mini cookie scoop will help keep them uniform. Makes roughly 20 balls (1 and 1/2 inch).
6. Place into fridge to set for at least an hour. Store in airtight container in fridge for up to 2 weeks or freezer for several months.

Prep Time: 15 Minutes

Cook Time: 15 Minutes

Servings: 5

Ingredients:

- 12 ounces gluten free pasta (I use THIS brand)
- 3 cups broccoli florets, divided
- 1/2 cup basil, parsley, or cilantro
- 1/2 cup olive oil (I use THIS organic, cold pressed brand)
- 1/3 cup pine nuts, pistachios, macadamia nuts, or pumpkin seeds
- Zest from 1/2 of a lemon
- 1 clove of garlic, peeled
- 1/2 tsp salt
- Extra olive oil, pine nuts, and fresh basil for garnish

Instructions

1. Cook the pasta in salted boiling water according to the package instructions until al dente.

2. Meanwhile, bring a medium pot of water to boil and place a bowl of ice water nearby. Blanch the broccoli florets in the boiling water for 30 seconds, dunk into the ice water to stop the cooking process, drain, and pat dry.

3. Place 2 cups of the blanched broccoli (save the remaining cup for later) into a food processor along with the basil, olive oil, pine nuts, lemon zest, garlic clove, and salt. Pulse until desired consistency. (I like mine super smooth.) Taste and adjust for salt and lemon zest.

4. To assemble: Transfer the hot cooked pasta to a serving bowl and top with broccoli pesto. Toss to combine. Add in remaining cup of blanched broccoli florets. Serve immediately, finished off with extra pine nuts, fresh basil, and a drizzle of olive oil. Store leftovers in an airtight container for 2-3 days.

Prep Time: 15 Minutes

Cook Time: 35 Minutes

Servings: 9

Ingredients:

The Filling:

- 2 cups fresh blueberries
- 1 tablespoon maple syrup
- 2 tsp arrowroot powder

The Crumble:

- 1 and 1/4 cup gluten free rolled oats
- 1 cup almond flour (I use THIS blanched brand)
- 1/4 cup finely chopped nuts (I used walnuts)
- 1 tsp baking powder
- 1/2 tsp salt
- 1/2 tsp cardamom (or cinnamon)
- 1/4 cup maple syrup
- 1/3 cup solid coconut oil (not melted)

Instructions

1. Preheat oven to 350'F. Liberally grease a 9 inch tart pan OR pie dish.
2. Toss blueberries in maple syrup and arrowroot powder until well combined. Set aside.
3. In a large bowl, stir together oats, almond flour, chopped nuts, baking powder, salt, and cardamom. Add is maple syrup and solid coconut oil. Use your fingers to massage the mixture until you get a coarse crumble.
4. Remove 3/4 cup of crumble to save for the topping. Press the remaining crumble firmly into prepared tart pan to make the crust. Spread blueberries evenly over crust and sprinkle on the reserved crumble topping.
5. Bake for 35-40 minutes, until crust is golden and filling is bubbling. Lay a piece of aluminum foil gently on top of pie for the last 15 minutes of baking to keep it from getting overly brown (almond flour likes to burn easily.)
6. Cool completely before slicing and serving.

Prep Time: 15 Minutes

Cook Time: 40 Minutes

Servings: 6

Ingredients:

- 2 tbsp ground flax seeds
- 5 tbsp warm water
- 1 and 1/4 cup mashed banana (about 3 ripe bananas)
- 1/4 cup coconut oil
- 1/3 cup maple syrup
- 2 tbsp coconut sugar
- 1 tsp vanilla extract
- 1 and 3/4 cups gluten free oat flour (see note)
- 1 and 1/2 tsp baking powder
- 1/2 tsp baking soda
- 1/2 tsp cardamom or cinnamon
- 1/2 tsp salt
- 1/3 cup chopped walnuts or pecans
- 1/3 cup chocolate chips (I use THESE sugar + dairy free kind)
- 1 cup raspberries

Instructions

1. To make flax eggs: whisk together 2 tablespoons of flax seed meal and 5 tablespoons of warm water and allow to sit for 10 minutes.

2. Preheat oven to 350'F. Line loaf pan with parchment paper.

3. In a large bowl, whisk together flax eggs, mashed banana, coconut oil, maple syrup, coconut sugar, and vanilla.

4. Add in oat flour, baking powder, baking soda, cardamom, and salt. Mix until just combined. Fold in walnuts and chocolate chips. And then carefully fold in raspberries. Pour the mixture into the lined loaf pan and bake for 50-60 minutes, until toothpick comes out clean in center. Loosely top with tin foil at 40 minute mark to keep top from over-browning.

5. Let loaf cool for 10 minutes then lift loaf out of pan to cool completely on a wire rack before slicing.

Prep Time: 15 Minutes

Cook Time: 20 Minutes

Servings: 10

Ingredients

- 2 tbsp flaxseed meal (see note)
- 5 tbsp warm water
- 1/3 cup coconut oil, melted
- 1/2 cup maple syrup
- 2 tbsp lemon juice
- Zest from 2 lemons
- 1 cup almond flour (I use THIS blanched brand)
- 1 cup gluten free oat flour
- 2 tsp baking powder
- 1 and 1/2 tbsp poppy seeds
- 1/4 tsp salt

For The Lemon Glaze:

- 1/4 cup coconut butter
- 1 tbsp coconut oil
- 1 tbsp maple syrup

- 1 tbsp lemon juice
- Hot water

Instructions

1. Make flax eggs: whisk together 2 tablespoons of flax seed meal and 5 tablespoons of warm water and allow to sit for 10 minutes.

2. Preheat oven to 350'F. Line muffin tray with muffin liners.

3. In a large bowl, whisk together prepared flax eggs, coconut oil, maple syrup, lemon juice, and lemon zest. Add in almond flour, oat flour, baking powder, poppy seeds, and salt. Mix until well incorporated.

4. Divide batter evenly among 8 to 10 muffin liners, depending on how big you like your muffins. Bake for 18-20 minutes, until golden and toothpick comes out clean in center.

5. When muffins are cool, prepare glaze by melting coconut butter and coconut oil in a small double boiler (I place a small glass bowl over a small pot). Whisk in 1 tablespoon of sweetener and lemon juice. Taste and add more sweetener if necessary. Don't worry if it gets clumpy. Remove from heat and whisk in hot water 1

teaspoon at a time until glaze is smooth and glossy. Keep whisking. It will get there.

6. Drizzle or spoon glaze over muffins. Garnish with extra lemon zest, if desired. ENJOY!

Prep Time: 15 Minutes

Cook Time: 35 Minutes

Servings: 9

Ingredients

For Blueberry Chia Jam:

- 3 cups blueberries
- 2 tbsp maple syrup
- 3 tbsp chia seeds

For Crumble Base:

- 2 cups gluten free rolled oats
- 1 cup almond flour (I use THIS blanched brand)
- 1/2 cup oat flour (like this OR grind your own)
- 1 tsp baking powder
- 1/4 tsp salt
- 1/2 tsp cardamom or cinnamon powder
- 1/2 tsp ginger powder
- 1/3 cup maple syrup
- 1/2 cup coconut oil, melted (or butter or ghee if not vegan)

Instructions

1. To make blueberry chia jam: add blueberries to a small sauce pan and cook over medium heat for 5 minutes, until berries begin to burst open. Add 2 tablespoons of maple syrup. With a fork or immersion blender, mash about half of the berries and simmer for another 5 minutes. Remove from heat and whisk in chia seeds until well incorporated. Set aside to cool and thicken.

2. Preheat oven to 350'F. Line 8×8 baking pan with parchment paper.

3. To make crumble: In a mixing bowl, combine oats, almond flour, oat flour, baking powder, salt, cardamom, and ginger. Stir in maple syrup and melted coconut oil until well incorporated.

4. To assemble: Press 2/3 of crumble mixture into bottom of prepared pan, packing it firmly and evenly. Spread blueberry jam in an even layer over the top of crumble base. Sprinkle remaining crumble mixture over the top.

5. Bake for 35-38 minutes, until crumble top is golden.

6. Remove from the oven and allow to cool to room temperature before slicing. Placing in refrigerator will speed cooling process.

7. Store any leftovers in air-tight container in the fridge.

Prep Time: 10 Minutes

Cook Time: 14 Minutes

Servings: 10

Ingredients:

- 1 tbsp ground flax seeds (flax meal)
- 3 tbsp warm water
- 1/4 cup peanut butter, almond butter, tahini, or sunflower butter
- 2 tbsp melted coconut oil or avocado oil
- 1 tsp vanilla extract
- 1 cup GF oats
- 1/4 cup GF oat flour (like this or grind your own)
- 1/3 cup coconut sugar
- 1/4 tsp salt
- Optional topping: coarse salt

Instructions

1. Make flax egg by whisking together 1 tablespoon of ground flax seeds and 3 tbsp warm water. Allow to sit for 10 minutes to gel.

2. Preheat oven to 350'F. Line baking sheet with parchment paper.

3. In a mixing bowl, whisk together flax egg, peanut butter, fat of choice, and vanilla until creamy smooth. Add rolled oats, oat flour, coconut sugar, and salt. Mix until well incorporated.

4. Using a small cookie scoop, drop small cookie balls onto prepared baking sheet. Flatten with fingers or fork to desired thickness. These cookies will not spread.

5. Bake for 12-14 minutes, until firm and golden on the bottom. Allow cookies to cool for 5 minutes on the baking tray then transfer to a wire rack to cool completely. Top with a bit of optional coarse salt while cooling.

Prep Time: 10 Minutes

Cook Time: 29 Minutes

Servings: 12

Ingredients

- 2 tbsp ground flax seeds see note
- 5 tbsp warm water
- 1 cup mashed ripe banana (2–3 bananas)
- 1/4 cup coconut oil, melted
- 1/2 cup maple syrup
- 1 tsp vanilla extract
- 1 cup almond flour (I use THIS blanched brand)
- 1 cup gluten free oat flour
- 1 cup gluten free oats
- 1 and 1/2 tsp baking powder
- 1/2 tsp baking soda
- 1/2 tsp cardamom or cinnamon
- 1/2 tsp salt
- Optional toppings: chopped walnuts and chocolate chips

Instructions

1. Stir together ground flax seed and warm water in a
    small bowl to make flax "eggs." Allow this mixture to
    sit and thicken for 10 minutes.
2. Preheat oven to 325'F. Line muffin tin with 12 paper
    muffin liners.
3. In a mixing bowl, whisk together flax eggs, mashed
    banana, coconut oil, maple syrup and vanilla until well
    incorporated.
4. Add almond flour, oat flour, oats, baking powder,
    baking soda, cardamom, and salt. Mix well until fully
    combined.
5. Divide batter evenly into 12 muffins liners. Top with
    optional chopped walnuts and chocolate chips... Bake
    for 27-29 minutes, until golden and toothpick comes
    out clean.
6. Cool on cooling rack. Enjoy!

11. Red Lentil Hummus

Prep Time: 5 Minutes

Cook Time: 20 Minutes

Servings: 2

Ingredients

- 1 and 1/2 cups water
- 1 cup red lentils, soaked for 4-8 hours (like this)
- 2 tbsp tahini (like this)
- 2 tbsp fresh lemon juice
- 1/4 tsp garlic powder OR 1 clove of garlic, peeled
- 2 tbsp olive oil
- Optional spices: cumin, smoked paprika
- Garnish: sesame seeds, fresh herbs, and more olive oil

Instructions

1. Bring one and half cups of water to a rolling boil in a small pot. Drain lentils and add to boiling water.

Reduce heat a bit and simmer until most of the liquid is absorbed and lentils are soft, about 20 minutes.

2. Remove lentils from heat and transfer to a glass bowl to cool for 10-15 minutes.

3. Add lentils, tahini, lemon juice, and garlic to food processor and process until creamy smooth, about 2 -3 minutes. Scrape down sides and add olive oil, salt to taste, and any optional spices. Process again until smooth. Adjust for salt and lemon.

4. Place in fridge to cool completely. It will thicken as it cools. Serve garnished with sesame seeds, fresh herbs, and an abundant drizzle of olive oil. Store in air-tight glass container in fridge for up to 5 days.

Prep Time: 10 Minutes

Cook Time: 17 Minutes

Servings: 12

Ingredients

- 2 cups almond flour (I use THIS blanched brand)
- 1/2 cup arrowroot powder (like this)
- 1 tsp baking soda
- 1/2 tsp salt
- 3 eggs
- 1/4 cup ghee, butter, or coconut oil, melted
- 1/3 cup maple syrup
- 2 tbsp fresh lemon juice
- Zest from one lemon
- 1 cup blueberries (plus more for sprinkling on top)

For The Lemon Glaze:

- 1/3 cup coconut butter (I use THIS brand)
- 1 tbsp coconut oil (I use THIS brand)
- 1–2 tbsp honey or maple syrup
- 1 tbsp fresh lemon juice

- hot water

Instructions

1. Preheat oven to 350'F. Line muffin tin with 12 paper liners.
2. Mix together almond flour, arrowroot, baking soda, and salt.
3. In another bowl, whisk together eggs, fat of choice, maple syrup, lemon juice, and zest. Add wet to dry and mix until well incorporated. Fold in blueberries.
4. Divide batter evenly into 12 muffin cups. Sprinkle a few blueberries on top of each muffin. Bake for 17-20 minutes, until golden on top and toothpick comes out clean in center. Remove from oven and allow to cool.
5. When muffins are cool, prepare glaze by melting coconut butter and coconut oil in a small double boiler (I place a small glass bowl over a small pot). Whisk in 1 tablespoon of sweetener and lemon juice. Taste and add more sweetener if necessary. Don't worry if it gets clumpy. Remove from heat and whisk in hot water 1 teaspoon at a time until glaze is smooth and glossy. Keep whisking. It will get there.
6. Drizzle glaze over muffins. ENJOY!

Prep Time: 15 Minutes

Cook Time: 40 Minutes

Servings: 9

Ingredients:

For Apple Topping:

- 1/2 cup apples, peeled and chopped
- 1 tbsp coconut sugar
- 1/2 tsp cinnamon powder

For Apple Cake Bars:

- 2 tbsp ground flax seeds
- 5 tbsp warm water
- 1 cup gluten free oat flour
- 3/4 cup almond flour
- 1 and 1/2 tsp baking powder
- 1/2 tsp baking soda
- 1 tsp cinnamon powder
- 1/4 tsp ginger powder
- 1/4 tsp cardamom or allspice
- 1/2 tsp salt

- 1/2 cup unsweetened apple sauce
- 1/4 cup coconut oil, melted
- 1/2 cup coconut sugar
- 1 tsp vanilla extract
- 1 cup apples, peeled and chopped

For Maple Glaze:

- 1/4 cup coconut butter
- 1 tbsp coconut oil
- 1 tbsp maple syrup
- Hot water

Instructions

1. Preheat oven to 350'F. Line an 8×8 pan with parchment paper.
2. To make apple topping, combine 1/2 cup chopped apples with coconut sugar and cinnamon. Set aside.
3. To make flax eggs, whisk together flax meal and warm water. Set aside for 5 minutes to gel.
4. In a medium bowl, combine oat flour, almond flour, baking powder, baking soda, spices, and salt.
5. In a large bowl. Whisk together apple sauce, coconut oil, coconut sugar, and vanilla extract. Whisk in flax

eggs. Add dry mixture to wet and stir until well incorporated. Fold in 1 cup of chopped apples.

6. Pour mixture into prepared baking pan. Spread apple topping over the top of mixture. Bake for 35-40 minutes until edges are golden and toothpick comes out clean in center.

7. Cool for 10 minutes in pan then then transfer to a wire rack to cool completely before adding maple glaze.

8. When apple bread bars are cool, prepare glaze by melting coconut butter and coconut oil in a small double boiler (I place a small glass bowl over a small pot). Whisk in 1 tablespoon of maple syrup. Taste and add more sweetener if necessary. Don't worry if it gets clumpy. Remove from heat and whisk in hot water 1 teaspoon at a time until glaze is smooth and glossy. Keep whisking. It will get there.

9. Once glaze is creamy, smooth, and thin enough to drip, drizzle or spoon over bars. Allow glaze to harden before cutting into 9 even-sized bars.

Prep Time: 5 Minutes

Cook Time: 25 Minutes

Servings: 5

Ingredients

- 1 cup mug dal (or red lentils) soaked for 4-8 hours
- 3/4 cup basmati rice (like this)
- 2 tbsp ghee or coconut oil
- 3/4 tsp mustard seeds (like this)
- 1 tsp cumin powder
- 5 cups of water, bone broth, or healing mineral broth
- 1–2 inch piece fresh ginger, peeled and grated
- 1/2 tsp turmeric powder
- 1/4 tsp ginger powder
- 1/4 tsp cardamom powder
- Salt to taste
- Fresh cilantro for garnish
- Ghee or coconut oil for drizzling

Instructions

1. Rinse both the soaked mug dal and rice very well and set aside.

2. Turn Instant Pot onto SAUTE mode and add 2 tbsp of ghee or coconut oil. When oil is hot, add mustard seeds and cumin powder and stir continually for about 1 minute until spices are fragrant. Be sure to not let them burn.

3. Pour in 5 cups of water or broth plus lentils, rice, fresh ginger, turmeric, ginger powder, and cardamom. Lock lid on IP and turn the vent valve to "sealing." Cook on HIGH pressure for 6 minutes. Allow to slow release for 10 minutes then release the pressure fully.

4. Add salt to taste. Stir in more water or broth if you prefer a soupier consistency. Serve immediately garnished with fresh cilantro and a dollop of ghee or coconut oil on top.

Prep Time: 5 Minutes

Cook Time: 25 Minutes

Servings: 6

Ingredients

- 2 tsp curry powder
- 1 tsp cumin powder
- 1 tsp turmeric powder
- 1/4 tsp garam masala
- Several grinds of black pepper
- 1/8 tsp cayenne (optional for some spice)
- 2 tbsp butter, ghee, of coconut oil
- 1 onion, chopped
- 3 cloves of garlic, minced
- 1 can full fat coconut milk (where to buy BPA free coconut milk)
- 1 cup broth (bone broth OR vegetable broth)
- 1/2 tsp salt
- 1 to 2 tsp fresh grated ginger (depending on how gingery you like it)
- 3 sweet potatoes (about 3 pounds)

- 1 small head of cauliflower (about 2 pounds)
- 2 pounds whole boneless, skinless chicken breasts
- 1 cup frozen green peas

Garnish:

- Fresh cilantro
- Lemon wedges

Instructions

1. In a small bowl, combine curry powder, turmeric, cumin, garam masala, pepper, and cayenne (if using.) Set aside.

2. Heat 2 tablespoons of fat of choice and saute onions until onions are translucent and starting to brown. Add garlic and spices and cook for another 30 seconds until spices are fragrant. Turn off heat and add in coconut milk, broth, ginger and salt. Stir to combine.

3. While onions cook, chop your sweet potatoes and cauliflower. Layer chicken breasts, sweet potatoes, and cauliflower in to slow cooker. Pour coconut milk mixture over top. Stir gently to combine.

4. Cook on high for 3-4 hours or low 6-7 hours. When cook time is done, remove chicken breasts from slow cooker. Set aside.

5. Add peas to slow cooker. Then shred chicken with 2 forks and add back to slow cooker. Cook for 5 minutes more.

6. Serve with fresh cilantro and lemon wedges.

Prep Time: 15 Minutes

Cook Time: 25 Minutes

Servings: 2

Ingredients:

- 1 small head of cauliflower
- 1 large sweet potato (or 2 small), chopped into small cubes
- 2 tbsp ghee, butter, or coconut oil, melted and divided
- 2 tsp turmeric powder (like this)
- 1/8 – 1/4 tsp cayenne powder (like this)
- Pinch of cinnamon powder (like this)
- 2 dried apricots, soaked in water for 5 minutes and chopped into small pieces.
- 2 eggs
- 2 cups packed of kale, DE stemmed and sliced into thin ribbons

Your favorite sauerkraut:

- 1 small beet, shredded

- Salt, pepper, and red pepper flakes for garnish

Creamy Turmeric Dressing:

- 1/4 cup tahini (like this)
- 3 tablespoon olive oil (I use THIS organic brand)
- 1 tablespoon lemon juice
- 1/4 cup water
- 1 tsp honey
- 1 1/2 tsp turmeric powder
- 1/4 tsp unrefined salt
- 2–3 pinches of black pepper

Instructions

1. Preheat oven to 425'F and bring a small pot of water to boil for eggs.
2. Remove the core from cauliflower and coarsely chop into florets, then place the cauliflower (in 2-3 batches) in a food processor and pulse until the cauliflower is small and has the texture of rice. Set aside.
3. Combine 1 tbsp of melted fat of choice with turmeric, cinnamon, and cayenne and pour over cauliflower rice. Mix to evenly coat. Spread evenly in a single layer onto baking sheet

4. Drizzle remaining 1 tablespoon of ghee/butter. Coconut oil over chopped sweet potatoes and spread evenly onto another baking sheet. Place both baking sheets in oven and bake for 25-30 minutes, flipping half way through, until golden. Toss is chopped apricots into cauliflower rice as it comes out of the oven.

5. While vegetables roast in oven, prepare greens, eggs and dressing. Once pot of water is boiling, gently place eggs into water and set timer for 6 minutes. Remove from water and place into cold water bath until ready to serve.

6. To prepare greens, steam kale until wilted but still bright green.

7. To prepare dressing, combine all ingredients in a small bowl and whisk until creamy smooth. Adjust for lemon, salt, and pepper.

8. To assemble comfort bowl, arrange roasted vegetables and kale into your favorite bowl. Add sauerkraut and shredded beets. Peel eggs, slice, and nest on top. Salt and pepper to taste. And red pepper flakes, if desired.

Prep Time: 2 Minutes

Cook Time: 5 Minutes

Servings: 1

Ingredients:

- 2 cups broccoli florets
- 1/2 cup basil, parsley, or cilantro
- 1/2 cup olive oil (I use THIS organic, cold pressed brand)
- 1/3 cup pine nuts, macadamia nuts, or pumpkin seeds
- Zest from half of a lemon
- 1/2 tsp salt

Optional:

- 1/2 tsp lemon juice
- 1 clove of garlic
- Pepper, to taste

Instructions

1. Fill a small glass bowl with ice water. Lightly steam broccoli florets for 3-4 minutes OR blanch in boiling water for 30 seconds. Then dunk into the ice water to stop the cooking process, drain, and pat dry.
2. Place cooled broccoli florets, basil (or parsley or cilantro), olive oil, pine nuts, lemon zest, and salt into food processor and pulse until desired consistency. (I like mine super smooth.) Taste and adjust for salt and lemon zest.
3. Store in air tight glass jar in fridge until ready to use.

Prep Time: 2 Minutes

Cook Time: 5 Minutes

Servings: 9

Ingredients:

- 1 medium zucchini, shredded
- Pinch of salt
- 1 and 1/2 large onions, halved and sliced into thin wedges
- 1 and 1/2 tbsp butter or ghee
- 1 pound asparagus
- 1 tsp butter, ghee, or coconut oil, melted
- 10 eggs
- 1/4 cup milk of any kind (I use THIS)
- 1 tsp salt
- 1/2 tsp garlic powder (like this)
- 1 tbsp fresh dill, finely chopped (or 1/2 tsp dried dill)
- Black pepper, to taste

For Garnish:

- Arugula

- Fresh dill

Instructions

1. Preheat oven to 400'F. Liberally oil a 9 inch cake pan and line bottom with a circle of parchment paper. Set aside.

2. Place grated zucchini in a colander, sprinkle with a pinch of salt, set aside in sink to drain.

3. To Make Caramelized Onions: Melt one and a half tablespoons of fat in a large skillet on medium heat. Add onions and cook for 30-35 minutes, stirring every few minutes. Reduce heat after about 20 minutes and stir more often. Reduce heat slightly and add a tablespoon of water if onions begin to stick or are getting too brown.

4. While onions cook, chop off woody ends of asparagus, arrange on a baking sheet, and drizzle on 1 tsp of melted fat, and roast in hot oven for 14 minutes, until spears begin to soften. Give the pan a shake halfway through. Remove from oven and allow to cool slightly. Reduce oven heat to 350'F.

5. Once onions are done, place shredded zucchini into a clean hand towel or a double layer of cheese cloth.

Squeeze excess moisture out to avoid a runny quiche. Roughly chop asparagus spears and place into prepared cake pan along with caramelized onions and squeezed zucchini. Gently mix to combine.

6. Whisk together eggs, milk, salt, garlic powder, dill, and pepper. Pour egg mixture over vegetables and shake pan to settle.

7. Bake at 350'F for 35-40 minutes, until center is set. Remove from oven and allow to cool slightly. Gently run a butter knife around the sides of cake pan and carefully invert quiche onto flat plate. Peel off parchment paper and invert the quiche one more time onto another plate to get the pretty side on top. Garnish and enjoy!

Prep Time: 10 Minutes

Cook Time: 10 Minutes

Servings: 4

Ingredients

For Creamy Poppy seed Dressing:

- 1/3 cup mayonnaise (homemade or THIS brand with healthy oils)
- 1/4 cup milk of any kind
- 2 tbsp olive oil (I use THIS organic brand)
- 1 tbsp apple cider vinegar (I use THIS raw brand)
- 1 tbsp fresh lemon juice
- 1 and 1/2 tsp poppy seeds
- 1 tsp honey or maple syrup (optional)
- Pinch of salt

For The Salad:

- 1 pound of chicken breast, cooked (see note on my favorite easy way to cook)
- 2–3 hard-boiled eggs, peeled and sliced

- 5 cups romaine lettuce, thinly sliced
- 1/2 cup of micro greens or sprouts
- 1 avocado, peeled and sliced
- 1 cup of blackberries
- 1 cup of blueberries
- 2 cups strawberries, sliced
- 1/4 cup pine nuts

Instructions

1. To make dressing: in a small bowl, whisk all dressing ingredients together until creamy smooth. Adjust for lemon flavor and salt. Set aside.
2. To assemble salad, arrange romaine and micro greens on a large platter. Add cooked chicken breast, sliced eggs, berries, avocado, and pine huts. Drizzle on dressing. Serve and enjoy!
3. Alternatively, you can plate romaine and micro greens on four individual plates and divide salad fixings evenly on top to make four individual servings. Drizzle dressing on top and serve.

Prep Time: 10 Minutes

Cook Time: 18 Minutes

Servings: 4

Ingredients:

Dressing:

- 1/2 cup good quality mayonnaise (homemade or THIS one)
- 1 tbsp lemon juice
- 2 tbsp water
- 1/2 tsp curry powder (like this)
- Salt and pepper, to taste

For Chicken Salad:

- 3 cups chopped chicken (leftover, rotisserie, or 2 medium cooked chicken breasts)
- 1/2 cup dried cranberries (I prefer fruit juice sweetened like THIS)
- 1 small apple – chopped
- 1 stalk celery- chopped
- 1/4 cup toasted pecans – chopped

Instructions

1. Whisk together all dressing ingredients in a small bowl. Adjust for lemon. Set aside.
2. Combine all chicken salad ingredients in a large bowl. Drizzle dressing over top and mix to combine.
3. Serve over crisp butter lettuce. Store leftovers in fridge for up to 3 days.

21. Thai Noodle Salad

Prep Time: 15 Minutes

Cook Time: 15 Minutes

Servings: 4

Ingredients

- 7 ounces pad Thai style rice noodles (like this) (or 3 cups of your fav veggie noodles)
- 3 cups shredded or grated cabbage (I used a mix of green and purple cabbage)
- 1 cup grated or julienned carrots
- 1 small red pepper, sliced
- 1/2 of a mango, peeled and chopped
- 1 packed cup fresh cilantro, roughly chopped
- 2 green onions, sliced
- 1/3 cup cashews, roughly chopped

Almond Butter Lime Dressing:

- 1/3 cup almond butter
- 1/3 cup lime juice

- 1/4 cup coconut amino (like this)

- 3 tbsp water

- 1–2 tsp honey or maple syrup

- 1 clove garlic

- a 2 inch knob of ginger, peeled and minced

- Splash of your fav hot sauce, optional

Instructions

1. Boil 4 cups of water in tea kettle or pot. Place rice noodles into a large glass bowl. Pour boiling water over noodles and allow to soften for about 10 minutes. Drain and rinse with cold water. Set aside.

2. Meanwhile, place all dressing ingredients into blender and process until creamy smooth. Adjust for sweetness and extra coconut amino, if desired. Thin with water, one tablespoon at a time, to get desired thickness. Set aside.

3. Chop, grate, and slice cabbage, carrots, red pepper, mango, and cilantro. Place cooled rice noodles into large bowl and add veggie mixture. Mix to combine. Top with green onions and cashews.

4. If serving entire salad, drizzle on dressing and toss until well coated. For individual servings, keep

undressed until ready to serve. Store leftovers of undressed salad for up to 4 days in fridge.

Prep Time: 5 Minutes

Cook Time: 10 Minutes

Servings: 8

Ingredients

- 1 pound ground turkey (I prefer ground thigh meat)
- 3/4 tsp salt
- 1 tbsp fresh sage, minced (or 1/2 tsp dried sage)
- 1/2 tsp dried thyme
- Black pepper, to taste
- 1 tbsp maple syrup (omit for WHOLE30)
- 1/2 cup fresh or frozen blueberries
- 1 tbsp butter, ghee, or coconut oil for cooking

Instructions

1. In a large bowl, combine turkey, salt, sage, thyme, pepper, and maple syrup until well incorporated. Gently fold in blueberries.
2. Roll into 8 even sized balls and gently flatten to about 1/2 inch thick.

3. Heat tablespoon of fat of choice in a large skillet on medium heat. Add in turkey patties and cook for about 4-5 minutes, until nice a brown on bottom. Flip and press down slightly to flatten a bit more. Cook for another 4 minutes, until cooked all the way through.

4. Enjoy! Leftovers can be stored in fridge for 2-3 days and frozen for several months. Simply reheat in toaster oven or oven in covered baking dish.

23. 5 Minute Avocado Salmon Salad

Prep Time: 5 Minutes

Cook Time: 5 Minutes

Servings: 2

Ingredients:

- 1 can of canned salmon (6 oz.) – drained (like this)
- 1/2 avocado – peeled and chopped
- 1 dill pickle – chopped
- 2 tbsp red onion, finely chopped
- 2 tbsp mayonnaise (homemade OR with avocado oil)
- 1 tbsp fresh herbs, finely chopped (I use cilantro but feel free to use parsley, basil, or dill)
- Salt and pepper – to taste

Instructions

1. Place all ingredients in a bowl and mix to combine. Add salt and pepper to taste.
2. Store in airtight container in fridge for up to 2 days.

Prep Time: 10 Minutes

Cook Time: 15 Minutes

Servings: 4

Ingredients

- 1 tbsp ghee, coconut oil, or avocado oil
- 2 cups butternut squash noodles
- 1/4 tsp salt
- 1/4 tsp garlic powder
- 2 eggs
- Extras: fresh herbs, sauerkraut, salad greens, red pepper flakes

Instructions

1. Melt fat of choice in a large skillet over medium heat. Add butternut squash noodles, salt, and garlic powder. Cook until noodles are tender but not falling apart – about 6-8 minutes. If noodles begin to stick, add a teaspoon or two of water.

2. Once noodles are tender, form into two nests with an indentation in the center. Crack an egg into center of each nest. Cook for 5-7 minutes, until whites are cooked but yolks are still soft. For more well done yolks, place lid onto skillet for a few minutes.

3. Use a spatula to transfer egg nests to a plate and add whatever extras you like: fresh herbs, sauerkraut, salad greens, red pepper flakes, etc.

Prep Time: 10 Minutes

Cook Time: 5 Minutes

Servings: 3

Ingredients

- 1 tbsp ghee, avocado oil, or coconut oil
- 2 cloves garlic, minced
- 4–5 medium zucchinis, cut into noodles
- 1 cup purple cabbage, shredded
- 1 cup carrots, shredded or julienned
- 1/4 cup coconut amino
- 2 tsp toasted sesame oil
- Juice from 1/2 of a lime
- 1 tbsp almond butter
- 1 tsp fresh ginger, grated
- Salt to taste
- Toasted sesame seeds for garnish

Instructions

1. Heat fat of choice in a large skillet over medium heat. Add garlic and cook for about 30 seconds. Stirring often. Add zucchini noodles, cabbage, and carrots. Cook for 3-5 minutes, until veggies are just tender. Use kitchen tongs to stir.

2. While the vegetables cook, whisk together coconut amino, toasted sesame oil, lime juice, almond butter, and ginger. Add salt to taste.

3. Once vegetables are tender, remove from heat and pour sesame ginger sauce over top. Toss to coat. Garnish with toasted sesame seeds and enjoy!

Prep Time: 10 Minutes

Cook Time: 6 Minutes

Servings: 2

Ingredients

- 2 flat breads (or one large flatbread pizza crust) (see above for suggestions)
- 1 tbsp butter, ghee, or avocado oil
- 4 cups baby spinach (about 5 ounces)
- 1/8 tsp garlic powder

Pinch of salt:

- 1/4 cup grated cheese like mozzarella, cheddar, or Gouda
- 2 tbsp grated parmesan cheese
- 1 oz. soft goat cheese
- 1–2 tbsp pine nuts

Instructions

1. Preheat oven to 400'F. Line baking sheet with parchment paper and set aside.

2. Heat fat of choice in large skillet and add in baby spinach. Saute for one minute and then add in garlic powder and pinch of salt. Cook for another minute, until spinach is wilted. Remove from heat.

3. Scatter cooked spinach evenly over flatbreads. Add grated cheese and parmesan. Then crumble goat cheese over the top. Add pine nuts.

4. Bake for 5-6 minutes, until flatbread is warm and starting to get crisp. Then broil for about a minute or two if you like the top a bit crispier. Enjoy!

Prep Time: 15 Minutes

Cook Time: 20 Minutes

Servings: 24

Ingredients

For Pesto:

- Bunch of basil (leaves only)
- 1 clove of garlic, peeled
- 1/4 cup pine nuts, macadamia nuts, hemp seeds, or pumpkin seeds
- 1/4 tsp salt
- 2 tbsp nutritional yeast (optional)
- 1/3 cup olive oil, plus more if needed (my fav organic brand)

For Meatballs:

- One pound ground chicken (thigh not breast)
- 1 egg
- 1/2 cup almond flour or cassava flour
- 1/4 cup pesto
- 1/2 tsp salt

Instructions

1. To make pesto: blend basil, garlic, pine nuts, salt, and optional nutritional yeast in food processor until you get a thick green paste. While processor is still running, slowly pour in olive oil. Scrape sides and add more olive oil until desire consistency is reached.

2. Preheat oven to 400' F. Line baking sheet with parchment paper OR place a cooling rack on top of baking sheet.

3. Combine all meatball ingredients in a large bowl until well incorporated.

4. Roll into 24 small meatballs (I use a small cookie scoop to get uniform balls) and place onto prepared baking sheet.

5. Bake for 18-20 minutes, until baked through and slightly golden. Be sure not to overcook.

6. Serve immediately with extra pesto drizzled on top. Meatballs freeze well for later use.

Prep Time: 10 Minutes

Cook Time: 10 Minutes

Servings: 24

Ingredients

- 3/4 cup natural peanut butter (like this)
- 1/4 cup plus 2 tbsp pumpkin puree (like this)
- 3 tbsp maple syrup (or honey)
- 1 tsp vanilla extract
- 1 tsp pumpkin pie spice (THIS is my fav brand)
- 1 and 1/2 cups gluten free rolled oats
- 1/4 cup flaxseed meal (like this) (or sub 1/4 cup almond flour)
- 2 tbsp chia seeds (I like THIS brand)
- 1/4 cup unsweetened shredded coconut
- 1/4 tsp salt
- 1/3 cup mini chocolate chips (I use THIS dairy and soy free brand)

Instructions

1. Whisk together peanut butter, pumpkin puree, maple syrup, vanilla extract, and pumpkin pie spice. Set aside.
2. In a food processor, pulse oats several times until broken up but not powdery. How chunky you want your oats is a personal preference.
3. Add oats, flaxseed meal, chia seeds, shredded coconut, and salt to peanut butter mixture. Mix to combine. Hands work best here. Fold in chocolate chips.
4. Roll into 24 balls. Using a mini ice cream scoop will help keep them uniform.
5. Store in air-tight container in fridge or freezer

Prep Time: 15 Minutes

Cook Time: 18 Minutes

Servings: 8

Ingredients

- 2 tbsp butter, ghee, or avocado oil
- 1 small onion, chopped
- 3 cloves garlic, minced
- 5 cups butternut squash, peeled and chopped
- 2 cup carrots, chopped
- 2 cups green lentils, rinsed and drained (like this)
- 8 cups broth (vegetable, homemade bone broth, or Kettle and Fire)
- 2 tsp Herpes de Provence (like this)
- 3 packed cups of kale, de-stemmed and chopped
- 1/4 cup parsley, chopped
- Salt and pepper to taste
- OPTIONAL: 1-2 tbsp lemon juice

Instructions

1. Turn Instant Pot to SAUTE and melt fat of choice. Saute onions until translucent, about 3-4 minutes. Add in garlic and cook another 30 seconds. Turn off IP.

2. Add in butternut squash, carrots, lentils, broth, and Herpes de Provence. Lock lid on IP and turn the vent valve to "sealing." Cook on HIGH pressure for 18 minutes then quick release the pressure. Turn off IP.

3. Remove 3-4 cups of soup, puree in blender, and add back to pot and stir to combine. Add in chopped kale and parsley, and close lid to let kale wilt and soften for a bit. Then salt and pepper to taste. For an added optional burst of flavor, add in a bit of fresh lemon juice. Enjoy!

Prep Time: 10 Minutes

Cook Time: 7 Minutes

Servings: 5

Ingredients

- 2 tbsp butter, ghee, coconut oil, or avocado oil
- 2 large leeks, trimmed, washed, and sliced
- 2 cloves garlic, minced
- 1 tbsp fresh ginger, grated
- 1 tsp turmeric powder (like this)
- 5 cups broccoli florets and stems, roughly chopped
- 4 cups cauliflower florets, roughly chopped
- 4 cups good quality broth (vegetable, homemade bone broth or Kettle and Fire)
- 1 tsp salt
- 1/8 tsp black pepper
- Optional: 1-2 tbsp fresh lemon juice

Instructions

1. Turn Instant Pot to SAUTE and melt fat of choice. Saute sliced leeks until they begin to soften, about 4-5 minutes. Add in garlic, ginger, and turmeric, and cook another minute. Turn off IP.

2. Add in broccoli, cauliflower, broth, and salt. Lock lid on IP and turn the vent valve to "sealing." Cook on HIGH pressure for 7 minutes then quick release the pressure. Turn off IP.

3. Add in black pepper and using an immersion hand blender (or regular blender), puree soup until creamy smooth. Taste and adjust for salt and pepper. Add in optional lemon juice for a bit of a flavor kick. Enjoy!